Low Carb Lifestyle

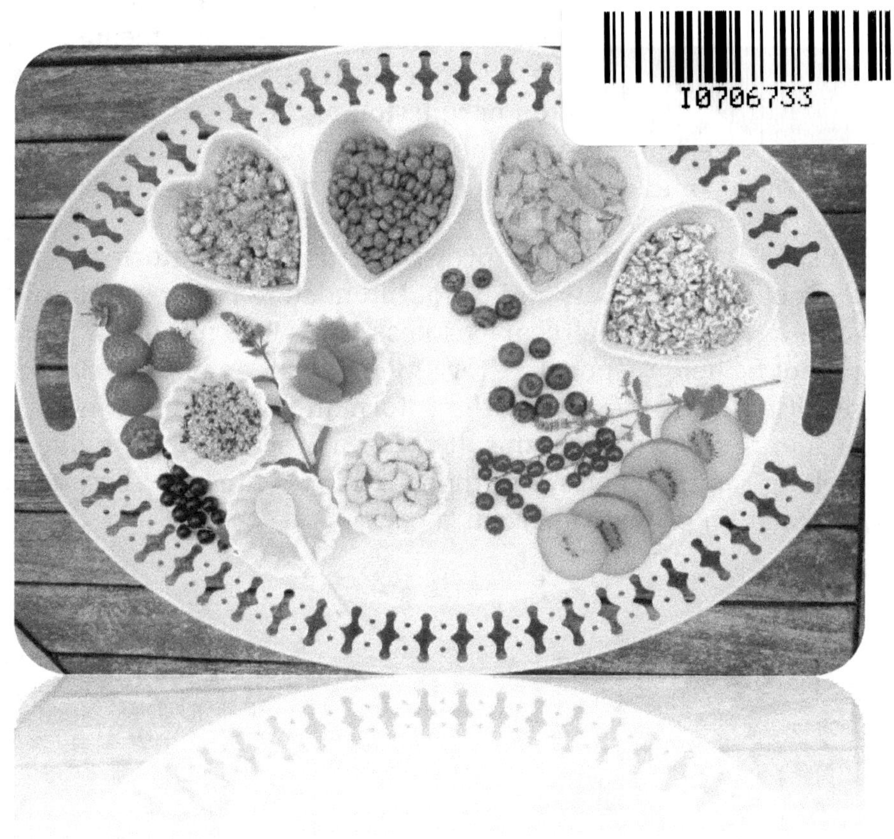

Low carb solution for weight management & health conditions

Mrs Sonali Chawadre

First Edition 2024

ISBN: 9798884942646

Copywrite

Copyright © [2024] by [Sonali Chawadre]

This book is intended to provide educational information on the topic of low carb diets and is not intended to replace medical advice from a qualified healthcare professional. The author and publisher cannot be held responsible for any personal or commercial damages resulting from the use of the information presented in this book. Readers are advised to consult with their healthcare provider before making any changes to their diet or lifestyle based on the information provided herein.

About the Author

Hello, I'm Sonali Chawadre, and I'm thrilled to share my expertise in clinical nutrition and dietetics with you. With a Master's degree in Clinical Nutrition and Dietetics, I've delved deep into the science of nutrition and its practical applications for promoting well-being.

My journey began in hospital settings, where I worked as a dedicated dietician, providing personalized dietary guidance to individuals with diverse health needs. Through this experience, I gained valuable insights into the challenges people face in maintaining a healthy lifestyle and developed effective strategies to overcome them.

Now, I'm excited to extend my reach beyond hospital walls by spreading knowledge through writing. With my debut book on low carb diets, I aim to empower you with the information and tools needed to make informed decisions about your health.

In my writing, I strive to make complex nutritional concepts easy to understand and apply in your daily life. My approach is grounded in evidence-based practices, ensuring that you can trust the information provided and make decisions backed by science.

I am passionate about promoting health and wellness, and I hope that my book serves as a valuable resource on your journey towards a healthier, happier life.

Preface

Welcome to the journey of discovering the power of low carb diets! In this book, we will explore how changing the way you eat can make a big difference in how you feel and your overall health.

We will break down the science behind low carb diets in simple terms, so you can understand why they work. From learning about different types of carbs to busting common myths, we will cover everything you need to know to make informed choices about your diet.

But this book is not just about facts—it is also a practical guide to help you put these ideas into action. You will find tips for meal planning, delicious recipes to try, and advice for dining out while sticking to your goals.

Whether you are just starting out on your low carb journey or looking for new ways to stay motivated, I am excited to share this journey with you. Together, let us discover the amazing benefits of low carb living and take steps towards a healthier, happier life.

Index

Introduction to Low Carb Diets

In recent years, low carb diets have gained immense popularity as a strategy for weight loss and overall health improvement. These diets, characterized by a reduction in carbohydrate intake while increasing consumption of protein and healthy fats, have been researched by various health experts and nutritionists. The fundamental principle underlying low carb diets is the restriction of carbohydrates, which are the body's primary source of energy. By reducing carb intake, the body is forced to burn stored fat for fuel, leading to weight loss and numerous other health benefits.

The concept of low carb diets traces back to the mid-19th century when William Banting, an English undertaker, popularized the idea of a low carbohydrate diet for weight loss in his pamphlet "Letter on Corpulence." However, it wasn't until the 20th century that low carb diets gained wider recognition with the advent of diets such as the Atkins Diet, the South Beach Diet, and the ketogenic diet.

The Atkins Diet, introduced by Dr. Robert Atkins in the 1970s, was one of the earliest low carb diets to gain mainstream attention. It emphasized the consumption of protein and fat while severely restricting carbohydrates, particularly refined sugars, and grains. The diet's popularity soared as individuals reported significant weight loss and improvements in various health markers.

Similarly, the ketogenic diet, initially developed in the 1920s as a treatment for epilepsy, gained renewed interest in recent years for its effectiveness in promoting weight loss and metabolic health. The ketogenic diet involves drastically reducing carbohydrate intake and increasing consumption of healthy fats, which induces a state of ketosis, wherein the body burns fat for fuel instead of carbohydrates.

The rationale behind low carb diets lies in their ability to regulate blood sugar levels and insulin secretion. Carbohydrates, especially refined sugars, and grains, are quickly broken down into glucose in the body, leading to rapid spikes in blood sugar and insulin levels. Over time, this continuous cycle of blood sugar spikes and insulin resistance can contribute to weight gain, inflammation, and various metabolic disorders.

By reducing carb intake, individuals can stabilize their blood sugar levels and improve insulin sensitivity, which is crucial for weight management and reducing the risk of chronic diseases such as type 2 diabetes and cardiovascular disease. Furthermore, low carb diets often lead to a reduction in appetite and cravings, making it easier for individuals to control their calorie intake and achieve sustainable weight loss.

One of the key misconceptions about low carb diets is that they promote the consumption of unhealthy fats and neglect the importance of fruits, vegetables, and whole grains. However low carb diets emphasize the importance of choosing nutrient-dense, whole foods such as leafy greens, non-starchy vegetables, lean proteins, nuts, seeds, and healthy fats like olive oil and avocado.

Low carb diets offer a compelling approach to weight loss and improved health by reducing carbohydrate intake and emphasizing nutrient-dense whole foods. While their efficacy and safety have been supported by numerous studies, its essential for individuals to consult with a healthcare professional before embarking on any dietary regimen, especially if they have underlying health conditions. In the subsequent chapters of this book, we will delve deeper into the science behind low carb diets, their potential benefits and risks, practical tips for implementation, and delicious recipes to support your journey towards better health and well-being.

The Science Behind Low Carb Diets and How They Work

Low carb diets have become increasingly popular in recent years, but what exactly is the science behind their effectiveness, and how do they work? To understand this, it is essential to delve into the metabolic processes that occur in the body in response to carbohydrate restriction.

Carbohydrates are the body's primary source of energy. When consumed, they are broken down into glucose, which is then used by the cells for fuel. However, excess glucose that is not immediately needed for energy is stored in the liver and muscles as glycogen. When glycogen stores are full, any additional glucose is converted into fat for long-term storage.

Low carb diets aim to reduce the intake of carbohydrates, thereby limiting the body's primary source of fuel. As a result, the body is forced to find alternative sources of energy, particularly stored fat. This metabolic state is known as ketosis.

Ketosis occurs when the body begins to break down fat into ketones, which can be used by the brain and other tissues for energy. Ketones are produced in the liver from fatty acids released from stored fat. In a state of ketosis, the body becomes more efficient at burning fat for fuel, leading to weight loss.

One of the key mechanisms by which low carb diets promote weight loss is through the regulation of insulin levels. Insulin is a hormone produced by the pancreas that helps regulate blood sugar levels by facilitating the uptake of glucose into cells. When carbohydrate intake is high, insulin levels spike to help transport glucose into cells for energy or storage. However, chronically elevated insulin levels can lead to insulin resistance, a condition associated with weight gain and metabolic disorders such as type 2 diabetes.

By reducing carbohydrate intake, low carb diets help stabilize blood sugar levels and lower insulin secretion. This not only promotes fat burning but also reduces hunger and cravings, making it easier for individuals to adhere to their dietary regimen and consume fewer calories overall.

Furthermore, low carb diets have been shown to have beneficial effects on various metabolic markers, including blood triglycerides, HDL cholesterol, and blood pressure. Studies have consistently demonstrated that low carb diets can lead to improvements in these markers, which are important for cardiovascular health.

Another aspect of the science behind low carb diets is their impact on appetite-regulating hormones. When carbohydrate intake is reduced, levels of ghrelin, the hunger hormone, tend to decrease, while levels of leptin, the satiety hormone, increase. This helps individuals feel fuller for longer periods, reducing the likelihood of overeating and promoting weight loss.

Moreover, low carb diets often lead to a greater loss of visceral fat, which is the type of fat that accumulates around organs in the abdominal cavity and is associated with an increased risk of chronic diseases such as heart disease and type 2 diabetes. By targeting visceral fat, low carb diets not only aid in weight loss but also improve metabolic health.

The science behind low carb diets revolves around their ability to induce ketosis, regulate insulin levels, reduce hunger and cravings, and improve metabolic health. By understanding these mechanisms, individuals can make informed choices about their dietary habits and harness the potential benefits of low carb eating for weight loss and overall health improvement. However, it is essential to consult with a healthcare professional before making any significant changes to your diet, especially if you have underlying health conditions.

Benefits of Low-Carb Eating for Weight Loss

Low-carb diets have significant attention for their effectiveness in promoting weight loss. By reducing carbohydrate intake and emphasizing protein and healthy fats, these diets offer several benefits that contribute to successful weight management.

One of the primary advantages of low-carb eating for weight loss is its ability to promote fat loss while preserving lean muscle mass. When carbohydrate intake is restricted, the body is forced to rely on stored fat for fuel, leading to a greater breakdown of fatty acids and ketone production. This metabolic state, known as ketosis, allows individuals to burn fat more efficiently, resulting in accelerated weight loss.

Moreover, low-carb diets have been shown to reduce appetite and cravings, making it easier for individuals to adhere to their dietary regimen and consume fewer calories overall. Studies have demonstrated that low-carb diets can lead to spontaneous reductions in calorie intake without the need for strict calorie counting or portion control. This is attributed to the satiating effects of protein and healthy fats, which help individuals feel fuller for longer periods and prevent overeating.

In addition to reducing calorie intake, low-carb diets have a positive impact on various metabolic markers associated with weight loss. Research has shown that low-carb diets can lead to improvements in insulin sensitivity, blood sugar control, and lipid profiles, all of which are important for managing weight and reducing the risk of chronic diseases such as type 2 diabetes and cardiovascular disease.

Furthermore, low-carb diets have been shown to target stubborn belly fat, which is particularly resistant to conventional weight loss methods. Visceral fat, the type of fat that accumulates around organs in the abdominal cavity, is metabolically active and associated with an increased risk of metabolic disorders. By reducing carbohydrate intake, low-carb diets promote the breakdown of visceral fat and improve metabolic health, leading to a reduction in waist circumference and abdominal obesity.

Another benefit of low-carb eating for weight loss is its flexibility and sustainability as a long-term dietary approach. Unlike restrictive fad diets that promote rapid weight loss through extreme calorie restriction or food elimination, low-carb diets allow individuals to enjoy a wide variety of foods while still achieving their weight loss goals. This flexibility makes it easier for individuals to adhere to their dietary regimen and maintain their results over time.

Moreover, low-carb diets offer numerous options for customization based on individual preferences and dietary needs. Whether someone prefers a moderate low-carb approach or a strict ketogenic diet, there are plenty of variations to suit different lifestyles and goals. This adaptability ensures that individuals can find a low-carb eating plan that works for them and fits seamlessly into their daily routine.

In conclusion, the benefits of low-carb eating for weight loss are numerous and well-supported by scientific research. From promoting fat loss and reducing appetite to improving metabolic health and offering long-term sustainability, low-carb diets offer a comprehensive approach to achieving and maintaining a healthy weight. However, it is important for individuals to consult with a healthcare professional before starting any new diet, especially if they have underlying health conditions or concerns. With proper guidance and support, low-carb eating can be an effective and enjoyable way to reach your weight loss goals and improve overall health and well-being.

Health Benefits Beyond Weight Loss: Improved Blood Sugar Control and Insulin Sensitivity

Low-carb diets offer more than just weight loss they provide significant health benefits too. By reducing carbohydrate intake, these diets enhance blood sugar control and insulin sensitivity, which are crucial for preventing and managing metabolic disorders like type 2 diabetes. This means that beyond weight management, low-carb eating supports improved regulation of blood sugar and insulin levels. When these factors are well-controlled, the risk of developing diabetes is reduced, and existing conditions can be managed more effectively. This underscores the broader health advantages of low-carb diets, highlighting their role in promoting overall well-being and reducing the risk of serious health issues associated with metabolic disorders.

When we consume carbohydrates, they are broken down into glucose, which enters the bloodstream and raises blood sugar levels. In response, the pancreas releases insulin, a hormone that helps transport glucose from the bloodstream into cells for energy or storage. However, in individuals with insulin resistance or impaired insulin sensitivity, the cells become less responsive to insulin, leading to elevated blood sugar levels and an increased risk of type 2 diabetes.

Low-carb diets help address this issue by reducing carbohydrate intake, thereby minimizing the fluctuations in blood sugar levels and insulin secretion. By consuming fewer carbohydrates, individuals experience smaller spikes in blood sugar after meals, which helps prevent insulin resistance and improve insulin sensitivity over time.

Numerous studies have demonstrated the effectiveness of low-carb diets in improving blood sugar control and insulin sensitivity. Research published in the American Journal of Clinical Nutrition found that individuals following a low-carb diet experienced greater improvements in insulin sensitivity compared to those on a low-fat diet, despite similar weight loss outcomes. Another study published in Diabetes Care showed that a low-carb diet led to significant reductions in fasting blood sugar levels and haemoglobin A1c (a marker of long-term blood sugar control) in individuals with type 2 diabetes.

Moreover, low-carb diets have been shown to be particularly beneficial for individuals with insulin resistance or prediabetes, a condition characterized by elevated blood sugar levels that are not yet high enough to be classified as type 2 diabetes. By reducing carbohydrate intake and promoting fat burning, low-carb diets help lower blood sugar levels and improve insulin sensitivity, thus reducing the risk of developing type 2 diabetes.

Beyond preventing diabetes, improved blood sugar control and insulin sensitivity have broader implications for overall health and well-being. Chronically elevated blood sugar levels and insulin resistance are associated with an increased risk of various metabolic disorders, including obesity, cardiovascular disease, and non-alcoholic fatty liver disease.

By stabilizing blood sugar levels and reducing insulin resistance, low-carb diets help mitigate these risks and improve metabolic health. Studies have shown that low-carb diets can lead to reductions in triglycerides, LDL cholesterol (the "bad" cholesterol), blood pressure, and markers of inflammation, all of which are important risk factors for cardiovascular disease.

Furthermore, improved blood sugar control and insulin sensitivity have been linked to other health benefits, including enhanced cognitive function, increased energy levels, and reduced risk of certain cancers. By optimizing metabolic health, low-carb diets support overall well-being and longevity, allowing individuals to enjoy a higher quality of life as they age.

The health benefits of low-carb eating extend far beyond weight loss, with improved blood sugar control and insulin sensitivity being among the most significant advantages. By reducing carbohydrate intake and promoting fat burning, low-carb diets help prevent and manage type 2 diabetes, as well as other metabolic disorders associated with insulin resistance. With proper guidance and support, incorporating low-carb eating into your lifestyle can lead to lasting improvements in health and vitality.

Insulin Sensitivity: Understanding its Importance and How to Improve It

Insulin sensitivity refers to the body's ability to respond efficiently to insulin, a hormone produced by the pancreas that helps regulate blood sugar levels. When cells are sensitive to insulin, they readily absorb glucose from the bloodstream in response to insulin secretion, leading to stable blood sugar levels and optimal energy utilization. However, when cells become resistant to insulin, as is the case in insulin resistance, they fail to respond adequately to insulin's signals, resulting in elevated blood sugar levels and a cascade of metabolic disturbances.

Maintaining optimal insulin sensitivity is crucial for overall health and well-being. When insulin sensitivity is impaired, the risk of developing type 2 diabetes, obesity, cardiovascular disease, and other metabolic disorders increases significantly. Therefore, understanding the factors that influence insulin sensitivity and implementing strategies to improve it are essential for promoting metabolic health and preventing chronic diseases.

Several factors can influence insulin sensitivity, including genetics, age, physical activity levels, dietary habits, and body composition. While some of these factors, such as genetics and age, are beyond our control, others, such as lifestyle choices and dietary patterns, can be modified to improve insulin sensitivity and overall metabolic health.

Regular physical activity is one of the most effective ways to enhance insulin sensitivity. Exercise increases glucose uptake by skeletal muscles, reduces liver glucose production, and enhances insulin signalling pathways, leading to improved insulin sensitivity. Both aerobic exercise, such as walking, jogging, and cycling, and resistance training, such as weightlifting and bodyweight exercises, have been shown to be beneficial for insulin sensitivity. Aim for at least 150 minutes of moderate-intensity aerobic activity or 75 minutes of vigorous-intensity aerobic activity per week, along with two days of strength training per week, to reap the metabolic benefits of exercise.

In addition to regular physical activity, dietary choices play a crucial role in modulating insulin sensitivity. Consuming a balanced diet rich in whole foods, including fruits, vegetables, whole grains, lean proteins, and healthy fats, can help improve insulin sensitivity and metabolic health. Avoiding processed foods, sugary beverages, refined carbohydrates, and excess saturated and trans fats is also important for maintaining optimal insulin sensitivity.

One dietary approach that has been shown to enhance insulin sensitivity is the low-carbohydrate diet. By reducing carbohydrate intake and emphasizing protein and healthy fats, low-carb diets help stabilize blood sugar levels, reduce insulin secretion, and promote fat burning, leading to improved insulin sensitivity. Studies have consistently demonstrated that low-carb diets can lead to significant improvements in insulin sensitivity, making them a valuable tool for preventing and managing insulin resistance and type 2 diabetes.

Furthermore, incorporating foods rich in specific nutrients known to support insulin sensitivity can further enhance metabolic health. For example, foods high in omega-3 fatty acids, such as fatty fish, flaxseeds, and walnuts, have been shown to improve insulin sensitivity and reduce inflammation. Similarly, consuming foods rich in magnesium, such as leafy greens, nuts, seeds, and whole grains, can help enhance insulin sensitivity and regulate blood sugar levels.

Insulin sensitivity plays a critical role in metabolic health, and maintaining optimal insulin sensitivity is essential for preventing and managing various chronic diseases. By incorporating regular physical activity, making healthy dietary choices, and implementing strategies such as low-carb eating and consuming nutrient-rich foods, individuals can improve insulin sensitivity and promote overall well-being. Working with a healthcare professional or registered dietitian can provide personalized guidance and support to optimize insulin sensitivity and achieve long-term metabolic health goals.

Misconceptions About Carbohydrates: Debunking Myths and Understanding the Truth

Carbohydrates have long been a topic of debate and controversy in the realm of nutrition. Despite being a fundamental source of energy for the body, carbohydrates have often been demonized and misunderstood. Here, we aim to debunk some of the most common misconceptions about carbohydrates and shed light on the truth behind these myths.

1. **Carbohydrates are inherently bad for health**: This is perhaps one of the most pervasive myths surrounding carbohydrates. While it is true that some carbohydrates, such as refined sugars and processed grains, can have negative health effects when consumed in excess, not all carbohydrates are created equal. In fact, many whole foods that are rich in carbohydrates, such as fruits, vegetables, legumes, and whole grains, are packed with essential nutrients, Fiber, and antioxidants that are beneficial for overall health.

2. **Carbohydrates cause weight gain**: Another common misconception is that carbohydrates are solely responsible for weight gain. While it is true that excessive consumption of refined carbohydrates and sugary foods can contribute to weight gain, the idea that all carbohydrates are fattening is inaccurate. In reality, weight gain is determined by an imbalance between calorie intake and expenditure, regardless of the macronutrient composition of the diet. Furthermore, complex carbohydrates, such as whole grains and starchy vegetables, can be part of a balanced diet and contribute to satiety and weight management when consumed in moderation.

3. **Carbohydrates should be eliminated for optimal health**: Some popular diet trends advocate for the complete elimination of carbohydrates, claiming that they are unnecessary and harmful to health. However, carbohydrates

are the body's primary source of energy, and they play a crucial role in fueling physical activity, supporting brain function, and maintaining overall metabolic health. Eliminating carbohydrates entirely can lead to nutrient deficiencies, low energy levels, and negative effects on mood and cognitive function.

4. **All carbohydrates are processed the same way in the body**: Another common misconception is that all carbohydrates are metabolized in the same way and have the same effect on blood sugar levels. Carbohydrates vary widely in their composition and impact on blood sugar. Simple carbohydrates, such as refined sugars and white bread, are quickly digested and can cause rapid spikes in blood sugar levels, while complex carbohydrates, such as whole grains and legumes, are digested more slowly, resulting in a more gradual rise in blood sugar and sustained energy release.

5. **Carbohydrates are addictive**: While it is true that many people crave and enjoy carbohydrate-rich foods, labelling carbohydrates as addictive oversimplifies the complex nature of food cravings and eating behaviours. Cravings for carbohydrates are often influenced by factors such as taste preferences, cultural influences, emotional triggers, and physiological hunger cues. Additionally, the idea of carbohydrate addiction lacks scientific evidence and fails to recognize the multifaceted nature of food intake and satiety regulation.

carbohydrates are an essential component of a balanced diet and play a crucial role in supporting overall health and well-being. While it is important to be mindful of the types and amounts of carbohydrates consumed, demonizing carbohydrates, and succumbing to common misconceptions can lead to unnecessary dietary restrictions and missed opportunities to enjoy nutritious and satisfying foods. By understanding the truth behind these myths and adopting a balanced approach to carbohydrate consumption, individuals can make informed choices that promote optimal health and vitality.

Choosing the Right Carbs: Understanding Glycemic Index and Glycemic Load

When it comes to carbohydrates, not all are created equal. The concept of glycemic index (GI) and glycemic load (GL) provides valuable insights into how different carbohydrate-containing foods affect blood sugar levels and overall health. By understanding these concepts, individuals can make informed choices about which carbs to include in their diet to promote stable blood sugar levels, sustained energy, and optimal health.

Glycemic Index (GI) is a measure of how quickly a carbohydrate-containing food raises blood sugar levels after consumption. Foods with a high GI value are rapidly digested and absorbed, leading to a rapid increase in blood sugar levels, while foods with a low GI value are digested more slowly, resulting in a gradual rise in blood sugar levels. The GI scale ranges from 0 to 100, with pure glucose having a GI value of 100.

Foods with a high GI value typically include refined carbohydrates, such as white bread, white rice, sugary snacks, and processed foods. These foods are quickly broken down into glucose in the body, leading to spikes in blood sugar levels and a corresponding insulin response. While high-GI foods can provide a quick source of energy, they often lead to a subsequent crash in energy levels and may contribute to weight gain, insulin resistance, and an increased risk of type 2 diabetes and cardiovascular disease.

On the other hand, foods with a low GI value are digested and absorbed more slowly, resulting in a more gradual rise in blood sugar levels and a sustained release of energy. Examples of low-GI foods include whole grains, legumes, fruits, vegetables, and nuts. These foods are rich in fiber, protein, and healthy fats, which help slow down the digestion and absorption of carbohydrates, leading to improved blood sugar control, increased satiety, and enhanced overall health.

Glycemic Load (GL) considers both the quantity and quality of carbohydrates in a serving of food, providing a more comprehensive measure of its impact on blood sugar levels. While GI indicates how quickly a food raises blood sugar levels, GL considers the actual amount of carbohydrates consumed in a typical serving size. This is important because even foods with a low GI value can have a high GL if consumed in large quantities.

To calculate the GL of a food, the GI value is multiplied by the amount of carbohydrates in a serving and divided by 100. Foods with a GL of 10 or less are considered low GL, while those with a GL of 20 or more are considered high GL.

By considering both GI and GL, individuals can make more informed choices about which carbohydrates to include in their diet to promote stable blood sugar levels and overall health. Choosing low-GI and low-GL foods, such as whole grains, legumes, fruits, vegetables, and nuts, can help prevent blood sugar spikes, reduce insulin resistance, and lower the risk of chronic diseases.

In summary, understanding glycemic index and glycemic load is essential for choosing the right carbohydrates to support optimal health and well-being. By focusing on low-GI and low-GL foods and incorporating them into a balanced diet, individuals can enjoy sustained energy levels, improved blood sugar control, and reduced risk of chronic diseases. Making informed choices about carbohydrate consumption is key to achieving and maintaining overall health and vitality.

Low Carb Meal Planning and Recipe Ideas

Embarking on a low carb diet does not mean sacrificing flavour or variety in your meals. With careful meal planning and creativity in the kitchen, you can enjoy a wide range of delicious and satisfying dishes while keeping your carbohydrate intake in check. Here, we will explore some practical tips for low carb meal planning and provide a variety of recipe ideas to inspire your culinary adventures.

Meal Planning Tips:

1. **Focus on Whole Foods:** Build your meals around nutrient-dense, whole foods that are naturally low in carbohydrates. These include non-starchy vegetables, leafy greens, lean proteins, and healthy fats. Incorporating a variety of colourful vegetables and lean proteins ensures that your meals are both nutritious and satisfying.

2. **Read Labels:** Pay attention to food labels and ingredient lists to identify hidden sources of carbohydrates, such as added sugars, refined grains, and starchy fillers. opt for minimally processed foods and choose products with the least amount of added sugars and refined carbohydrates.

3. **Plan:** Take time to plan your meals for the week ahead, considering your schedule, dietary preferences, and nutritional goals. This can help you stay organized, save time and money, and avoid last-minute temptations to stray from your low carb eating plan.

4. **Batch Cooking:** Prepare large batches of low carb staples, such as grilled chicken, roasted vegetables, and quinoa, to use as building blocks for multiple meals throughout the week. This simplifies meal prep and allows for easy customization and variety in your meals.

5. **Experiment with Substitutions:** Get creative in the kitchen by experimenting with low carb substitutions for high carb ingredients. For example, cauliflower can be used as a

substitute for rice or mashed potatoes, zucchini noodles (zoodles) can replace traditional pasta, and lettuce wraps for tortillas or bread.

Now, let us explore some delicious low carb recipe ideas to inspire your meal planning:

Breakfast:

1. **Spinach and Feta Omelette:** Whisk together eggs and pour into a hot skillet. Add sautéed spinach and crumbled feta cheese. Cook until set, then fold the omelette in half and serve with sliced avocado on the side.

2. **Low Carb Smoothie:** Blend together spinach, avocado, unsweetened almond milk, protein powder, and a handful of berries for a refreshing and nutrient-packed breakfast option.

Lunch:

1. **Grilled Chicken Caesar Salad:** Top a layer of romaine lettuce with grilled chicken breast, put some Parmesan cheese, and a creamy Caesar dressing made with Greek yogurt.

2. **Turkey and Avocado Lettuce Wraps:** Fill large lettuce leaves with sliced turkey breast, avocado, sliced tomato, and crispy bacon for a satisfying and portable lunch option.

Dinner:

1. **Zucchini Noodles with Pesto and Cherry Tomatoes:** Spiralize zucchini into noodles and sauté in olive oil until tender. Toss with homemade pesto sauce and halved cherry tomatoes for a light and flavourful pasta alternative.

2. **Grilled Salmon with Asparagus:** Marinate salmon fillets in a mixture of lemon juice, garlic, and herbs, then grill until

cooked through. Serve alongside roasted asparagus drizzled with olive oil.

3. **Stuffed Bell Peppers:** Cut bell peppers in half and remove seeds. Fill with a mixture of cooked ground turkey, cauliflower rice, diced tomatoes, onions, and spices. Bake until peppers are tender and filling is heated through.

<u>Snacks:</u>

1. **Celery Sticks with Almond Butter:** Spread almond butter on celery sticks for a crunchy and satisfying snack that is packed with protein and healthy fats.

2. **Cheese and Veggie Platter:** Arrange slices of cheese, cucumber, bell peppers, and cherry tomatoes on a platter for a colourful and nutritious snack option.

With these meal planning tips and recipe ideas, you will be well-equipped to enjoy a delicious and satisfying low carb diet that supports your health and wellness goals. Whether you are looking to lose weight, improve metabolic health, or simply adopt a more balanced eating pattern, low carb eating can be both enjoyable and sustainable with the right approach and mindset.

Tips for Dining Out on a Low Carb Diet

Dining out can present challenges for individuals following a low carb diet, as many restaurant menus are dominated by carb-heavy dishes. However, with some planning and savvy decision-making, it is entirely possible to enjoy a satisfying and delicious meal while sticking to your low carb eating plan. Here are some tips to help you navigate dining out on a low carb diet:

1. **Research the Menu in Advance:** Before heading to a restaurant, look at the menu online if possible. Look for low carb options such as grilled meats, seafood, salads, and vegetable-based dishes. Many restaurants now offer gluten-free or keto-friendly menus, making it easier to identify suitable options.

2. **Choose Protein-Rich Foods:** opt for protein-rich dishes such as grilled chicken, steak, fish, or tofu as the main component of your meal. Protein not only helps keep you feeling full and satisfied but also provides essential nutrients for muscle repair and maintenance.

3. **Swap Carbs for Vegetables:** When ordering a meal, ask if you can substitute carb-heavy sides such as potatoes, rice, or bread for extra vegetables or a side salad. Most restaurants are willing to accommodate special requests, so do not be afraid to ask for customization to suit your dietary needs.

4. **Be Mindful of Hidden Carbs:** Be aware of hidden sources of carbohydrates in restaurant dishes, such as sauces, dressings, and marinades. Ask for sauces and dressings on the side so you can control the amount you consume, or request substitutions for lower carb options like olive oil and vinegar.

5. **Skip the Bread Basket:** Resist the temptation to indulge in bread or breadsticks offered before the meal arrives. Instead, focus on enjoying a protein-rich appetizer or a salad with a low carb dressing to start your meal on the right foot.

6. **Choose Grilled or Baked Options:** opts for grilled, baked, or roasted dishes instead of fried or breaded items, which tend to be higher in carbs. Grilled meats and seafood are flavourful and satisfying choices that align well with a low carb eating plan.

7. **Watch Portion Sizes:** Restaurant portions are often larger than what you might typically eat at home, so consider sharing an entree with a dining companion or asking for a half portion if available. Alternatively, you can ask for a to-go box upfront and save half of your meal for later.

8. **Stay Hydrated:** Drink plenty of water throughout your meal to help fill you up and prevent overeating. Avoid sugary beverages like soda and fruit juices, and opt for unsweetened options such as water, sparkling water, or herbal tea instead.

9. **Practice Moderation with Alcohol:** If you choose to enjoy an alcoholic beverage with your meal, be mindful of its carb content. Stick to dry wines, spirits, or light beers, and limit your intake to one or two servings to minimize the impact on your blood sugar levels.

10. **Focus on Enjoying the Experience:** Lastly, remember that dining out is not just about the food it is also about the experience of socializing and enjoying time with friends and family. Focus on the company and conversation rather than fixating on food, and do not stress too much if you can't find the perfect low carb option. Making the best choice you can in the moment is what matters most.

By following these tips and strategies, you can navigate dining out on a low carb diet with confidence and ease. With a little planning and flexibility, you can enjoy delicious meals while staying true to your dietary goals and priorities.

Overcoming Challenges and Staying Motivated on a Low Carb Diet

Starting and sticking to a low carb diet can be challenging, especially in a world where carbohydrate-rich foods are abundant and often highly tempting. However, with the right mindset, strategies, and support, it is entirely possible to overcome these challenges and stay motivated on your low carb journey. Here are some common obstacles faced by individuals following a low carb diet and tips for staying motivated:

1. **Cravings for Carbohydrates:** One of the most significant challenges of a low carb diet is dealing with cravings for carbohydrate-rich foods like bread, pasta, and sweets. These cravings can be intense, especially during the initial phase of transitioning to a low carb eating plan. To overcome cravings, focus on incorporating satisfying and flavourful low carb alternatives into your meals, such as vegetables, lean proteins, and healthy fats. Experiment with different recipes and cooking techniques to keep your meals exciting and satisfying without feeling deprived.

2. **Social Pressures and Temptations:** Dining out, attending social gatherings, and navigating family events can present challenges for individuals following a low carb diet. It's common to face pressure from others to indulge in carb-heavy foods or to feel left out when everyone else is enjoying their favourite dishes. To stay motivated in social settings, communicate your dietary preferences and goals with friends and family members, and do not be afraid to advocate for yourself. Look for low carb options on menus or offer to bring a dish that aligns with your dietary needs to social gatherings.

3. **Plateauing Weight Loss:** While many people experience rapid weight loss when first starting a low carb diet, it is common to hit a plateau or experience slower progress over time. Plateaus can be frustrating and demotivating, but they

are a normal part of the weight loss journey. To break through a plateau and stay motivated, focus on other indicators of progress besides the scale, such as improvements in energy levels, mood, and overall well-being. Experiment with different meal plans, exercise routines, and lifestyle changes to keep your body guessing and jumpstart your progress.

4. **Limited Food Choices:** Following a low carb diet may initially feel restrictive, especially if you are used to relying heavily on carbohydrate-rich foods. However, with a little creativity and experimentation, you can discover a wide variety of delicious low carb options to enjoy. Focus on incorporating a diverse array of whole foods into your diet, including vegetables, fruits, nuts, seeds, lean meats, poultry, fish, and dairy products. Explore different cuisines and cooking methods to keep your meals interesting and satisfying.

5. **Lack of Support:** Maintaining motivation on a low carb diet can be challenging without a strong support system. If your friends, family, or coworkers do not understand or support your dietary choices, it can feel isolating and discouraging. Seek out support from like-minded individuals, whether online or in-person, who can provide encouragement, accountability, and practical tips for success. Joining a low carb community, participating in forums or social media groups, or enlisting the help of a supportive friend or family member can make a world of difference in staying motivated on your low carb journey.

6. **Negative Self-Talk:** It is easy to fall into the trap of negative self-talk and self-criticism when faced with challenges or setbacks on a low carb diet. Instead of beating yourself up for slip-ups or perceived failures, practice self-compassion and kindness towards yourself. Focus on the progress you have made, no matter how small, and celebrate your successes along the way. Remember that change takes time and effort,

and setbacks are a natural part of the process. By cultivating a positive mindset and practicing self-care, you can stay motivated and resilient in the face of challenges on your low carb journey.

Staying motivated on a low carb diet requires patience, perseverance, and a positive mindset. By acknowledging and addressing common challenges, seeking out support, and focusing on the benefits of a low carb lifestyle, you can overcome obstacles and achieve your health and wellness goals. Remember that every step forward, no matter how small, brings you closer to success, and that with determination and commitment, you can thrive on your low carb journey.

Incorporating Exercise into a Low Carb Lifestyle

Exercise is an essential component of a healthy lifestyle, and when combined with a low carb diet, it can enhance weight loss, improve metabolic health, and boost overall well-being. However, navigating the relationship between exercise and low carb eating can sometimes be challenging. Here, we will explore some tips and strategies for effectively incorporating exercise into a low carb lifestyle:

1. **Choose the Right Type of Exercise:** When following a low carb diet, it is important to select exercises that complement your dietary goals and preferences. Focus on incorporating a combination of cardiovascular exercise, strength training, and flexibility exercises into your routine for optimal results. Cardiovascular activities such as walking, running, cycling, and swimming help burn calories and improve cardiovascular health, while strength training exercises such as weightlifting and bodyweight exercises help build lean muscle mass and boost metabolism. Flexibility exercises such as yoga and stretching can improve mobility and reduce the risk of injury.

2. **Fuel Your Workouts Appropriately:** While it is common to rely on carbohydrates for energy during exercise, individuals following a low carb diet may need to adjust their approach to fueling workouts. Since glycogen stores may be lower on a low carb diet, it is important to prioritize protein and healthy fats as sources of energy before and after exercise. Consider consuming a small snack or meal containing protein and healthy fats, such as Greek yogurt with nuts or a protein shake with avocado, before a workout to provide sustained energy and support muscle recovery.

3. **Stay Hydrated:** Proper hydration is essential for optimal exercise performance and recovery, regardless of your dietary preferences. Drink plenty of water before, during, and after exercise to replace fluids lost through sweat and

prevent dehydration. Consider adding electrolytes to your water, especially if you are engaging in prolonged or intense exercise, to maintain electrolyte balance and prevent muscle cramps.

4. **Monitor Your Energy Levels:** Pay attention to how your body responds to exercise on a low carb diet and adjust your approach accordingly. Some individuals may find that they have lower energy levels during workouts when first starting a low carb diet, while others may experience increased stamina and endurance over time. Listen to your body's signals and adjust the intensity and duration of your workouts as needed to ensure that you are able to perform at your best while still adhering to your low carb eating plan.

5. **Focus on Recovery:** Proper recovery is essential for maximizing the benefits of exercise and minimizing the risk of injury. Make sure to prioritize rest and recovery days in your exercise routine to allow your body time to repair and rebuild muscle tissue. Incorporate recovery strategies such as foam rolling, stretching, and massage to alleviate muscle soreness and improve flexibility. Additionally, prioritize quality sleep and nutrition to support your body's recovery process and promote overall well-being.

6. **Be Patient and Persistent:** Like any lifestyle change, incorporating exercise into a low carb lifestyle takes time, patience, and persistence. Don't expect to see overnight results, and be prepared to adjust your routine as needed based on your individual needs and preferences. Focus on the long-term benefits of regular exercise, such as improved fitness, strength, and energy levels, rather than short-term weight loss goals.

Incorporating exercise into a low carb lifestyle is both feasible and beneficial for achieving and maintaining optimal health and well-being. By choosing the right type of exercise, fueling your workouts appropriately, staying hydrated, monitoring your energy levels, focusing on recovery, and being patient and persistent, you can successfully integrate exercise into your low carb lifestyle and reap the numerous benefits it has to offer. Remember that consistency is key, and that by making exercise a priority in your daily routine, you can achieve your fitness and wellness goals while enjoying the many advantages of a low carb lifestyle.

Potential Risks and Side Effects of Low Carb Diets

While low carb diets have gained popularity for their effectiveness in promoting weight loss and improving metabolic health, it is important to recognize that they may not be suitable for everyone and can come with potential risks and side effects. Understanding these risks can help individuals make informed decisions about whether a low carb diet is right for them and how to mitigate potential negative consequences. Here, we will explore some of the potential risks and side effects of low carb diets:

1. **Nutrient Deficiencies:** One of the primary concerns with low carb diets is the risk of nutrient deficiencies. By restricting carbohydrate-rich foods such as fruits, grains, and legumes, individuals may inadvertently limit their intake of essential vitamins, minerals, and fiber. Deficiencies in nutrients such as vitamin C, potassium, magnesium, and fiber can lead to symptoms such as fatigue, weakness, constipation, and impaired immune function. To mitigate this risk, it is important to prioritize nutrient-dense, whole foods and consider incorporating supplements if needed.

2. **Keto Flu:** When transitioning to a low carb diet, some individuals may experience symptoms commonly referred to as "keto flu." These symptoms, which can include fatigue, headache, nausea, dizziness, and irritability, typically occur during the initial phase of carbohydrate restriction as the body adjusts to using fat for fuel instead of carbohydrates. While keto flu is usually temporary and resolves within a few days to weeks, it can be uncomfortable and may deter some individuals from sticking to their low carb eating plan.

3. **Digestive Issues:** Low carb diets, particularly those high in animal proteins and fats, can sometimes lead to digestive issues such as constipation, diarrhoea, and bloating. This may be due to changes in gut microbiota, reduced fiber intake, or inadequate hydration. To alleviate digestive discomfort,

individuals following a low carb diet should prioritize fiber-rich vegetables, stay hydrated, and consider incorporating probiotic-rich foods such as yogurt or fermented vegetables into their diet.

4. **Increased Risk of Heart Disease:** While low carb diets have been shown to improve certain cardiovascular risk factors such as blood sugar levels, triglycerides, and HDL cholesterol, some research suggests that they may also increase the risk of heart disease in the long term. This is particularly true for low carb diets that are high in saturated fats and low in Fiber-rich foods. To minimize the risk of heart disease, individuals following a low carb diet should focus on consuming healthy fats such as monounsaturated and polyunsaturated fats, and prioritize whole foods over processed and refined foods.

5. **Potential for Muscle Loss:** In some cases, very low carb diets, particularly those that severely restrict protein intake, may lead to muscle loss over time. This can occur when the body breaks down muscle tissue for energy in the absence of sufficient dietary protein and carbohydrates. To preserve muscle mass on a low carb diet, it's important to consume an adequate amount of protein and engage in regular strength training exercises to stimulate muscle growth and repair.

6. **Disordered Eating Patterns:** For some individuals, the strict rules and restrictions of a low carb diet may trigger disordered eating patterns such as orthorexia, binge eating, or obsessive food tracking. This can lead to feelings of guilt, anxiety, and preoccupation with food, as well as negative impacts on mental health and overall well-being. To prevent disordered eating behaviours, it's important to approach low carb diets with a balanced and flexible mindset, and to prioritize self-care, mindfulness, and intuitive eating practices.

Low carb diets can be effective for weight loss and improving metabolic health, they are not without potential risks and side effects. It is important for individuals considering a low carb diet to weigh the potential benefits against the potential risks and to approach dietary changes with caution and awareness. Consulting with a healthcare professional or registered dietitian can provide personalized guidance and support to ensure that a low carb diet is safe and appropriate for individual needs and goals. Additionally, focusing on a balanced and sustainable approach to eating, prioritizing nutrient-dense foods, and listening to your body's signals can help mitigate potential negative consequences and promote overall health and well-being.

Low Carb Diet and Mental Health: Mood and Cognitive Function

While low carb diets are primarily known for their impact on weight loss and metabolic health, emerging research suggests that they may also have implications for mental health, including mood regulation and cognitive function. Here, we will explore the relationship between low carb diets and mental health, focusing on their potential effects on mood and cognitive function:

1. **Stabilizing Blood Sugar Levels:** One of the key mechanisms by which low carb diets may impact mental health is through their ability to stabilize blood sugar levels. By reducing the consumption of high Glycemic carbohydrates, which can lead to rapid spikes and crashes in blood sugar levels, low carb diets help maintain more stable and consistent energy levels throughout the day. This can have a positive effect on mood regulation, as fluctuations in blood sugar levels have been linked to changes in mood, including irritability, anxiety, and depression.

2. **Increased Availability of Ketones:** Another potential mechanism by which low carb diets may influence mental health is through the increased production of ketones, which are produced by the liver when carbohydrate intake is restricted. Ketones serve as an alternative fuel source for the brain, providing a steady supply of energy even when glucose levels are low. Some research suggests that ketones may have neuroprotective effects and may enhance cognitive function and mood stability. However, more research is needed to fully understand the role of ketones in mental health.

3. **Reduced Inflammation:** Low carb diets are often rich in anti-inflammatory foods such as vegetables, fruits, nuts, seeds, and healthy fats, while also reducing the intake of pro-inflammatory foods such as refined sugars and grains. Chronic inflammation has been implicated in the

development of mood disorders such as depression and anxiety, as well as cognitive decline and neurodegenerative diseases. By reducing inflammation in the body, low carb diets may help support mental health and cognitive function.

4. **Improved Brain Health:** Some studies suggest that low carb diets may promote the production of brain-derived neurotrophic factor (BDNF), a protein that plays a key role in promoting the growth, survival, and plasticity of neurons in the brain. Higher levels of BDNF have been associated with improved mood, cognitive function, and resilience to stress. Additionally, low carb diets may support brain health by reducing oxidative stress and promoting the production of neurotransmitters such as serotonin and dopamine, which play important roles in mood regulation and cognitive function.

5. **Potential Challenges:** While low carb diets may offer benefits for mental health, it is important to note that they may not be suitable for everyone, and some individuals may experience negative effects on mood and cognitive function when first starting a low carb diet. This may be due to factors such as carbohydrate withdrawal symptoms, changes in gut microbiota, or nutrient deficiencies. It is important to listen to your body's signals and adjust your dietary approach as needed to ensure that it supports both your physical and mental health.

low carb diets have the potential to impact mental health in various ways, including mood regulation and cognitive function. By stabilizing blood sugar levels, increasing the availability of ketones, reducing inflammation, supporting brain health, and promoting overall well-being, low carb diets may offer benefits for mental health beyond their effects on weight loss and metabolic health. However, it is important to approach dietary changes with caution and awareness, and to prioritize a balanced and sustainable approach to eating that supports both physical and mental health. Consulting with a healthcare professional or registered dietitian can provide personalized guidance and support to ensure that a low carb diet is safe and appropriate for individual needs and goals.

Low Carb Diet for Specific Health Conditions: Diabetes, PCOS, and Metabolic Syndrome

Low carb diets have gained recognition not only for their effectiveness in promoting weight loss but also for their potential therapeutic benefits in managing certain health conditions. In particular, low carb diets have shown promise in improving outcomes for individuals with diabetes, polycystic ovary syndrome (PCOS), and metabolic syndrome. Here, we will explore how low carb diets can be tailored to address the unique needs of these specific health conditions:

1. **Diabetes:** Low carb diets are increasingly recognized as a valuable dietary approach for managing diabetes, particularly type 2 diabetes. By reducing carbohydrate intake and moderating blood sugar levels, low carb diets can help improve Glycemic control and reduce the need for insulin or other diabetes medications. Research has shown that low carb diets can lead to significant improvements in HbA1c levels, fasting blood sugar levels, and insulin sensitivity in individuals with diabetes. Additionally, low carb diets may help reduce the risk of complications associated with diabetes, such as cardiovascular disease and kidney damage.

When following a low carb diet for diabetes management, it is important to focus on whole, nutrient-dense foods such as non-starchy vegetables, lean proteins, healthy fats, and low Glycemic index fruits. Monitoring carbohydrate intake, portion sizes, and blood sugar levels is essential for optimizing Glycemic control and preventing hypoglycaemia. Consulting with a healthcare professional or registered dietitian who specializes in diabetes management can provide personalized guidance and support to ensure that a low carb diet is safe and effective for individual needs and goals.

2. **Polycystic Ovary Syndrome (PCOS):** PCOS is a hormonal disorder characterized by insulin resistance, irregular menstrual cycles, and symptoms such as acne, hirsutism

(excessive hair growth), and infertility. Low carb diets have shown promise in improving insulin sensitivity, reducing insulin levels, and promoting weight loss in women with PCOS. By reducing carbohydrate intake and moderating insulin levels, low carb diets can help address the underlying hormonal imbalances associated with PCOS and improve symptoms such as irregular periods, acne, and excess hair growth.

When following a low carb diet for PCOS management, it is important to focus on whole, unprocessed foods and avoid sugary and refined carbohydrates. Emphasizing high-fibers foods such as vegetables, fruits, legumes, and whole grains can help promote satiety, stabilize blood sugar levels, and support hormonal balance. Incorporating regular physical activity, managing stress levels, and prioritizing adequate sleep are also important components of a holistic approach to managing PCOS symptoms.

3. **Metabolic Syndrome:** Metabolic syndrome is a cluster of conditions that occur together, including abdominal obesity, high blood pressure, high blood sugar levels, and abnormal lipid levels (e.g., high triglycerides, low HDL cholesterol). It significantly increases the risk of cardiovascular disease, type 2 diabetes, and other chronic health problems. Low carb diets have been shown to be effective in improving several components of metabolic syndrome, including reducing abdominal fat, lowering blood pressure, improving insulin sensitivity, and improving lipid profiles.

When following a low carb diet for managing metabolic syndrome, it is important to focus on reducing carbohydrate intake, particularly refined sugars and grains, while emphasizing whole, nutrient-dense foods. Prioritizing sources of healthy fats such as avocados, nuts, seeds, and olive oil can help improve lipid profiles and promote heart health. Regular physical activity, stress management, and smoking cessation are also important lifestyle factors for managing metabolic syndrome and reducing cardiovascular risk.

low carb diets can be valuable dietary approaches for managing specific health conditions such as diabetes, PCOS, and metabolic syndrome. By reducing carbohydrate intake and focusing on whole, nutrient-dense foods, low carb diets can help improve Glycemic control, hormone balance, and metabolic health, leading to better outcomes and reduced risk of complications. However, it is important for individuals with these health conditions to work closely with healthcare professionals or registered dietitians to ensure that a low carb diet is safe and appropriate for their individual needs and goals. With proper guidance and support, low carb diets can be powerful tools for improving health and well-being in individuals with diabetes, PCOS, and metabolic syndrome.

Sustainability and Long-Term Success with a Low Carb Lifestyle

The popularity of low carb diets has surged in recent years, with many individuals adopting this dietary approach for weight loss, improved metabolic health, and overall well-being. However, for a dietary pattern to be truly sustainable and effective in the long term, it must be practical, flexible, and enjoyable, allowing individuals to maintain their health goals while still enjoying a fulfilling lifestyle. In this chapter, we will explore the principles of sustainability and long-term success with a low carb lifestyle, including strategies for overcoming common challenges and maintaining motivation over time.

<u>Understanding Sustainability in the Context of a Low Carb Lifestyle:</u>

Sustainability refers to the ability to maintain a behaviour or lifestyle pattern over the long term, without experiencing significant negative consequences or detracting from overall well-being. When it comes to a low carb lifestyle, sustainability encompasses several key factors:

1. **Nutritional Adequacy:** A sustainable low carb lifestyle should provide all the essential nutrients needed for optimal health and well-being. This means focusing on nutrient-dense foods such as vegetables, fruits, lean proteins, healthy fats, and whole grains (if tolerated), while minimizing the intake of processed and refined carbohydrates. Adequate intake of vitamins, minerals, and other essential nutrients is essential for supporting overall health and preventing nutrient deficiencies.

2. **Practicality and Convenience:** A sustainable low carb lifestyle should be practical and convenient for everyday life. This means choosing foods that are readily available, easy to prepare, and enjoyable to eat. It also involves finding practical solutions for dining out, traveling, and socializing while still adhering to a low carb eating plan. By

incorporating flexibility and adaptability into their approach, individuals can make sustainable choices that fit their lifestyle and preferences.

3. **Health Benefits:** A sustainable low carb lifestyle should provide tangible health benefits that contribute to long-term well-being. This may include improvements in weight management, metabolic health, blood sugar control, cardiovascular health, and overall vitality. By focusing on long-term health outcomes rather than short-term weight loss goals, individuals can stay motivated and committed to their low carb lifestyle over time.

4. **Psychological Well-being:** A sustainable low carb lifestyle should also support psychological well-being by promoting a positive relationship with food, body image, and self-care. This involves cultivating a mindset of self-compassion, mindfulness, and moderation, rather than restriction or deprivation. By fostering a healthy attitude towards food and nourishing both body and mind, individuals can sustainably maintain their low carb lifestyle while also enjoying life's pleasures.

<u>Strategies for Long-Term Success with a Low Carb Lifestyle:</u>

Achieving long-term success with a low carb lifestyle requires a combination of practical strategies, psychological resilience, and social support. Here are some tips for maintaining sustainability and achieving lasting results:

1. **Focus on Whole, Nutrient-Dense Foods:** Emphasize whole, nutrient-dense foods such as vegetables, fruits, lean proteins, and healthy fats in your low carb eating plan. These foods provide essential nutrients, fibers, and antioxidants that support overall health and well-being.

2. **Experiment with Different Food Choices:** Keep your low carb lifestyle interesting and enjoyable by experimenting with a variety of foods, Flavors, and recipes. Explore new

ingredients, cooking techniques, and cuisines to keep meals exciting and satisfying.

3. **Plan and Be Prepared:** Take time to plan your meals and snacks for the week ahead, and stock your kitchen with low carb staples foods such as vegetables, protein sources, nuts, seeds, and healthy fats. Having healthy options readily available makes it easier to stick to your low carb eating plan, even on busy days routine.

4. **Stay Hydrated:** Drink plenty of water throughout the day to stay hydrated and support overall health and well-being. Hydration is especially important on a low carb diet, as it can help prevent constipation, support digestion, and promote satiety.

5. **Listen to Your Body:** Pay attention to your body's hunger and fullness cues, and eat mindfully to avoid overeating. Practice intuitive eating by tuning into your body's signals and eating in response to physical hunger rather than emotional cues.

6. **Manage Stress:** Incorporate stress-reducing activities such as meditation, yoga, deep breathing exercises, or time in nature into your daily routine to promote relaxation and mental well-being. Chronic stress can negatively impact both physical and mental health, so it is important to prioritize stress management as part of your low carb lifestyle.

7. **Seek Support:** Surround yourself with supportive friends, family members, or online communities who share your health goals and can provide encouragement, and motivated. Having support network can make it easier to stay on track with your low carb lifestyle and overcome challenges along the way.

8. **Be Flexible and Forgiving:** Remember that no one is perfect, and it is normal to have occasional slip-ups or

setbacks on your low carb journey. Be kind to yourself and practice self-compassion when things do not go as planned. Instead of dwelling on mistakes, focus on making positive choices moving forward and learning from your experiences.

Achieving sustainability and long-term success with a low carb lifestyle requires a holistic approach that prioritizes nutritional adequacy, practicality, health benefits, and psychological well-being. By focusing on whole, nutrient-dense foods, experimenting with different food choices, planning, staying hydrated, listening to your body, managing stress, seeking support, and being flexible and forgiving, individuals can maintain a low carb lifestyle that supports their health goals and enhances their overall quality of life. With dedication, perseverance, and a positive mindset, a low carb lifestyle can be not only effective but also enjoyable and sustainable for the long term.